PROSTATE CANCER

Causes, Symptoms, Signs, Diagnosis, Treatments, Stages. What You Need to Know About Prostate Cancer

National Cancer Institute (Author), U.S. Department of Health and Human Services (Author), National Institutes of Health (Author), S.Smith (Editor)

Prostate Cancer

Table of Contents

About This Booklet

This National Cancer Institute (NCI) booklet is about cancer* of the prostate. Each year, more than 186,000 American men learn they have this disease. Prostate cancer is the second most common type of cancer among men in this country. Only skin cancer is more common.

Learning about medical care for prostate cancer can help you take an active part in making choices about your care. This booklet tells about:

- Diagnosis and staging
- Treatment options
- Tests you may have after treatment
- Taking part in research studies

This booklet has lists of questions that you may want to ask your doctor. Many people find it helpful to take a list of questions to a doctor visit. To help remember what your doctor says, you can take notes or ask whether you may use a tape recorder. You may also want to have a family member or friend go with you when you talk with the doctor—to take notes, ask questions, or just listen.

For the latest information about prostate cancer, please visit our Web site at http://www.cancer.gov/ cancertopics/types/prostate. Or, contact our Cancer Information Service. We can answer your questions about cancer. We can also send you NCI booklets and fact sheets. Call 1–800–4–CANCER (1–800–422–6237) or instant message us through the LiveHelp service at http://www.cancer.gov/help.

*Words in italics are in the Dictionary on page 35. The Dictionary explains these terms. It also shows how to pronounce them.

The Prostate

The prostate is part of a man's reproductive system. It's an organ located in front of the rectum and under the bladder. The prostate surrounds the urethra, the tube through which urine flows.

A healthy prostate is about the size of a walnut. If the prostate grows too large, it squeezes the urethra. This may slow or stop the flow of urine from the bladder to the penis.

The prostate is a gland. It makes part of the seminal fluid. During ejaculation, the seminal fluid helps carry sperm out of the man's body as part of semen.

Male hormones (androgens) make the prostate grow. The testicles are the main source of male hormones, including testosterone. The adrenal gland also makes testosterone, but in small amounts.

Prostate Cancer Cells

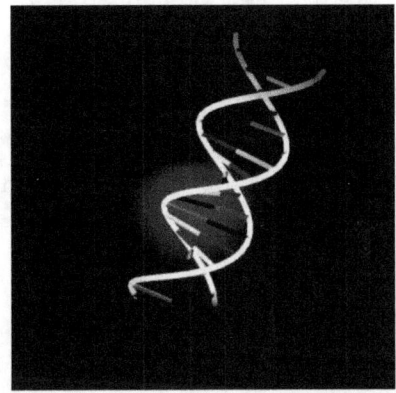

Cancer begins in cells, the building blocks that make up tissues. Tissues make up the organs of the body.

Normal cells grow and divide to form new cells as the body needs them. When normal cells grow old or get damaged, they die, and new cells take their place.

Sometimes, this process goes wrong. New cells form when the body doesn't need them, and old or damaged cells don't die as they should. The buildup of extra cells often forms a mass of tissue called a growth or tumor.

Prostate growths can be benign (not cancer) or malignant (cancer).

Benign prostatic hyperplasia (BPH) is a benign growth of prostate cells. It is not cancer. The prostate grows larger and squeezes the urethra. This prevents the normal flow of urine.

BPH is a very common problem. In the United States, most men over the age of 50 have symptoms of BPH. For some men, the symptoms may be severe enough to need treatment.

To learn about BPH and other prostate changes that are not cancer, read NCI's booklet

Understanding Prostate Changes: A Health Guide for Men.

Benign growths are not as harmful as malignant growths:
- Benign growths (such as BPH):
—are rarely a threat to life
—can be removed and probably won't grow back — don't invade the tissues around them

—don't spread to other parts of the body
- Malignant tumors:
—may be a threat to life
—often can be removed, but sometimes grow back
—can invade and damage nearby tissues and organs
—can spread to other parts of the body

Cancer cells can spread by breaking away from the prostate tumor. They enter blood vessels or lymph vessels, which branch into all the tissues of the body. The cancer cells can attach to other tissues and grow to form new tumors that may damage those tissues. The spread of cancer is called metastasis. See the Staging section on page 12 for information about prostate cancer that has spread.

Risk Factors

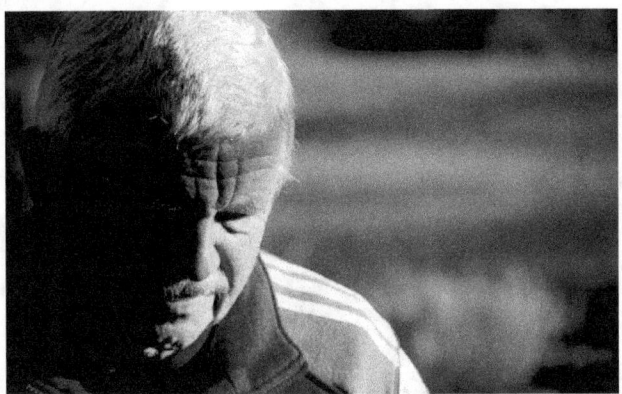

When you're told you have prostate cancer, it's natural to wonder what may have caused the disease. But no one knows the exact causes of prostate cancer. Doctors seldom know why one man develops prostate cancer and another doesn't.

However, research has shown that men with certain risk factors are more likely than others to develop prostate cancer. A risk factor is something that may increase the chance of getting a disease.

Studies have found the following risk factors for prostate cancer:

• Age over 65: Age is the main risk factor for prostate cancer. The chance of getting prostate cancer increases as you get older. In the United States, most men with prostate cancer are over 65. This disease is rare in men under 45.

• Family history: Your risk is higher if your father, brother, or son had prostate cancer.

• Race: Prostate cancer is more common among black men than white or Hispanic/Latino men. It's less common among Asian/Pacific Islander and American Indian/Alaska Native men.

• Certain prostate changes: Men with cells called high-grade prostatic intraepithelial neoplasia (PIN) may be at increased risk of prostate cancer. These prostate cells look abnormal under a microscope.

• Certain genome changes: Researchers have found specific regions on certain chromosomes that are linked to the risk of prostate cancer. According to recent studies, if a man has a genetic change in one or more of these regions, the risk of prostate cancer may be increased. The risk increases with the number of genetic changes that are found. Also, other studies have shown an elevated risk of prostate cancer among men with changes in certain genes, such as BRCA1 and BRCA2.

Having a risk factor doesn't mean that a man will develop prostate cancer. Most men who have risk factors never develop the disease.

Many other possible risk factors are under study. For example, researchers have studied whether vasectomy (surgery to cut or tie off the tubes that carry sperm out of the testicles) may pose a risk, but most studies have found no increased risk. Also, most studies have shown that the chance of getting prostate cancer is not increased by tobacco or alcohol use, BPH, a sexually transmitted disease, obesity, a lack of exercise, or a diet high in animal fat or meat. Researchers continue to study these and other possible risk factors.

Researchers are also studying how prostate cancer may be prevented. For example, they are studying the possible benefits of certain drugs, vitamin E, selenium, green tea extract, and other substances. These studies are with men who have not yet developed prostate cancer.

Symptoms

A man with prostate cancer may not have any symptoms. For men who do have symptoms, the common symptoms include:

- Urinary problems
—Not being able to pass urine

—Having a hard time starting or stopping the urine flow

—Needing to urinate often, especially at night —Weak flow of urine

—Urine flow that starts and stops

—Pain or burning during urination

- Difficulty having an erection
- Blood in the urine or semen
- Frequent pain in the lower back, hips, or upper thighs

Most often, these symptoms are not due to cancer. BPH, an infection, or another health problem may cause them. If you have any of these symptoms, you should tell your doctor so that problems can be diagnosed and treated.

Detection and Diagnosis

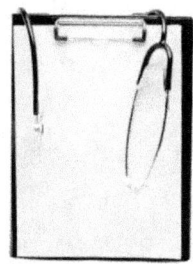

Your doctor can check for prostate cancer before you have any symptoms. During an office visit, your doctor will ask about your personal and family medical history. You'll have a physical exam. You may also have one or both of the following tests:

• Digital rectal exam: Your doctor inserts a lubricated, gloved finger into the rectum and feels your prostate through the rectal wall. Your prostate is checked for hard or lumpy areas.

• Blood test for prostate-specific antigen (PSA): A lab checks the level of PSA in your blood sample. The prostate makes PSA. A high PSA level is commonly caused by BPH or prostatitis (inflammation of the prostate). Prostate cancer may also cause a high PSA level. See the NCI fact sheet The Prostate-Specific Antigen (PSA) Test: Questions and Answers.

The digital rectal exam and PSA test are being studied in clinical trials to learn whether finding prostate cancer early can lower the number of deaths from this disease.

The digital rectal exam and PSA test can detect a problem in the prostate. However, they can't show whether the problem is cancer or a less serious condition. If you have abnormal test results, your doctor may suggest other tests to make a diagnosis. For example, your visit may include other lab tests, such as a urine test to check for blood or infection. Your doctor may order other procedures:

- Transrectal ultrasound: The doctor inserts a probe

into the rectum to check your prostate for abnormal areas. The probe sends out sound waves that people cannot hear (ultrasound). The waves bounce off the prostate. A computer uses the echoes to create a picture called a sonogram.

- Transrectal biopsy: A biopsy is the removal of tissue to look for cancer cells. It's the only sure way to diagnose prostate cancer. The doctor inserts needles through the rectum into the prostate. The doctor removes small tissue samples (called cores) from many areas of the prostate. Transrectal ultrasound is usually used to guide the insertion of the needles. A pathologist checks the tissue samples for cancer cells.

You may want to ask the doctor these questions before having a transrectal ultrasound or biopsy:

• Where will the procedure take place? Will I have to go to the hospital?

• How long will it take? Will I be awake?

• Will it hurt? Will I need local anesthesia?

• What are the risks? What are the chances of infection or bleeding afterward?

• How do I prepare for it? Will I need to avoid taking aspirin to reduce the chance of bleeding? Will I need an enema before the procedure?

• How long will it take me to recover? Will I be given an antibiotic or other medicine afterward?

• How soon will I know the results? If a biopsy is done, will I get a copy of the pathology report?

• If I do have cancer, who will talk to me about the next steps? When?

If Cancer Is Not Found

If cancer cells are not found in the biopsy sample, ask your doctor how often you should have checkups. Information about BPH and other benign prostate problems can be found in the NCI booklet

Understanding Prostate Changes: A Health Guide for Men.

If Cancer Is Found

If cancer cells are found, the pathologist studies tissue samples from the prostate under a microscope to report the grade of the tumor. The grade tells how much the tumor tissue differs from normal prostate tissue. It suggests how fast the tumor is likely to grow.

Tumors with higher grades tend to grow faster than those with lower grades. They are also more likely to spread. Doctors use tumor grade along with your age and other factors to suggest treatment options.

One system of grading is with the Gleason score. Gleason scores range from 2 to 10. To come up with the Gleason score, the pathologist uses a microscope to look at the patterns of cells in the prostate tissue. The most common pattern is given a grade of 1 (most like normal cells) to 5 (most abnormal).

If there is a second most common pattern, the pathologist gives it a grade of 1 to 5, and adds the two most common grades together to make the Gleason score. If only one pattern is seen, the pathologist counts it twice. For example, 5 + 5 = 10. A high Gleason score (such as 10) means a high-grade prostate tumor. High-grade tumors are more likely than low-grade tumors to grow quickly and spread.

Another system of grading prostate cancer uses grades 1 through 4 (G1 to G4). G4 is more likely than G1, G2, or G3 to grow quickly and spread.

For more about tumor grade, see the NCI fact sheet Tumor Grade: Questions and Answers.

Staging

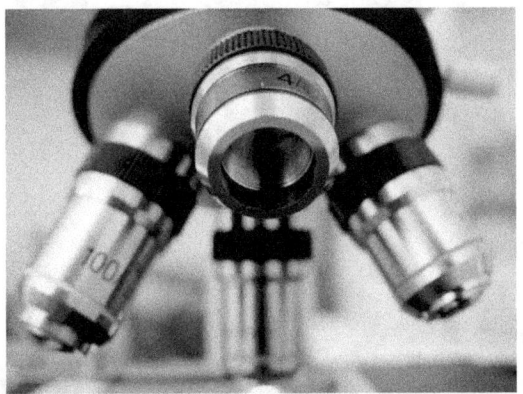

If the biopsy shows that you have cancer, your doctor needs to learn the extent (stage) of the disease to help you choose the best treatment. Staging is a careful attempt to find out whether the tumor has invaded nearby tissues, whether the cancer has spread and, if so, to what parts of the body.

Some men may need tests that make pictures of the body:

• Bone scan: The doctor injects a small amount of a radioactive substance into a blood vessel. It travels through the bloodstream and collects in the bones. A machine called a scanner detects and measures the radiation. The scanner makes pictures of the bones on a computer screen or on film. The pictures may show cancer that has spread to the bones.

• CT scan: An x-ray machine linked to a computer takes a series of detailed pictures of your pelvis or other parts of the body. Doctors use CT scans to look for prostate cancer that has spread to lymph nodes and other areas. You may receive contrast material by injection into a blood vessel in your arm or hand, or by enema. The contrast material makes abnormal areas easier to see.

• MRI: A strong magnet linked to a computer is used to make detailed pictures of areas inside your body. The doctor can view these pictures on a monitor and can print them on film. An MRI can show whether cancer has spread to lymph nodes or other areas. Sometimes contrast material makes abnormal areas show up more clearly on the picture.

When prostate cancer spreads, it's often found in nearby lymph nodes. If cancer has reached these nodes, it also may have spread to other lymph nodes, the bones, or other organs.

When cancer spreads from its original place to another part of the body, the new tumor has the same kind of abnormal cells and the same name as the primary tumor. For example, if prostate cancer spreads to bones, the cancer cells in the bones are actually prostate cancer cells. The disease is metastatic prostate cancer, not bone cancer. For that reason, it's treated as prostate cancer, not bone cancer. Doctors call the new tumor "distant" or metastatic disease.

These are the stages of prostate cancer:

• Stage I: The cancer can't be felt during a digital rectal exam, and it can't be seen on a sonogram. It's found by chance when surgery is done for another reason, usually for BPH. The cancer is only in the prostate. The grade is G1, or the Gleason score is no higher than 4.

• Stage II: The tumor is more advanced or a higher grade than Stage I, but the tumor doesn't extend beyond the prostate. It may be felt during a digital rectal exam, or it may be seen on a sonogram.

• Stage III: The tumor extends beyond the prostate. The tumor may have invaded the seminal vesicles, but cancer cells haven't spread to the lymph nodes.

• Stage IV: The tumor may have invaded the bladder, rectum, or nearby structures (beyond the seminal vesicles). It may have spread to the lymph nodes, bones, or to other parts of the body.

Treatment

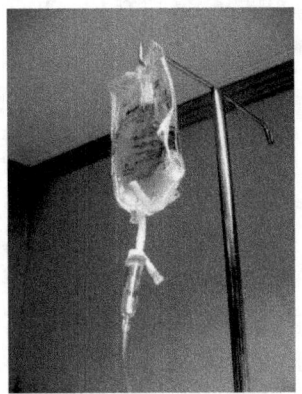

Men with prostate cancer have many treatment options. The treatment that's best for one man may not be best for another. The options include active surveillance (also called watchful waiting), surgery, radiation therapy, hormone therapy, and chemoYou may have a combination of treatments.

The treatment that's right for you depends mainly on your age, the grade of the tumor (the Gleason score), the number of biopsy tissue samples that contain cancer cells, the stage of the cancer, your symptoms, and your general health. Your doctor can describe your treatment choices, the expected results of each, and the possible side effects. You and your doctor can work together to develop a treatment plan that meets your medical and personal needs.

You may want to talk to your doctor about taking part in a clinical trial, a research study of new treatment methods. See the section on Taking Part in Cancer Research on page 32.

Your doctor may refer you to a specialist, or you may ask for a referral. You may want to see a urologist, a surgeon who specializes in treating problems in the urinary or male sex organs. Other specialists who treat prostate cancer include urologic oncologists, medical oncologists, and radiation oncologists. Your health care team may also include an oncology nurse and a registered dietitian.

Before treatment starts, ask your health care team about possible side effects and how treatment may change your normal activities. For example, you may want to discuss with your doctor the possible effects on sexual activity. The NCI booklet Treatment Choices for Men with Early-Stage Prostate Cancer can tell you more about treatments and their side effects.

At any stage of the disease, supportive care is available to relieve the side effects of treatment, to control pain and other symptoms, and to help you cope with the feelings that a diagnosis of cancer can bring. You can get information about coping on the NCI Web site at http://www.cancer.gov/

cancertopics/coping and from NCI's Cancer Information Service at 1–800–4–CANCER or LiveHelp (http://www.cancer.gov/help).

questions before choosing your treatment:

- What is the grade of the tumor?
- What is the stage of the disease? Has the cancer spread? Do any lymph nodes show signs of cancer?

- What is the goal of treatment? What are my treatment choices? Which do you recommend for me? Why?

- What are the expected benefits of each type of treatment?
- What are the risks and possible side effects of each treatment? How can side effects be managed?

- What can I do to prepare for treatment?
- Will I need to stay in the hospital? If so, for how long?
- How will treatment affect my normal activities? Will it affect my sex life? Will I have urinary problems? Will I have bowel problems?

- What will the treatment cost? Will my insurance cover it?

- Would a clinical trial (research study) be appropriate for me?
- Can you recommend other doctors who could give me a second opinion about my treatment options?

Active Surveillance

You may choose active surveillance if the risks and possible side effects of treatment outweigh the possible benefits. Your doctor may suggest active surveillance if you're diagnosed with early stage prostate cancer that seems to be slowly growing. Your doctor may also offer this option if you are older or have other serious health problems.

Choosing active surveillance doesn't mean you're giving up. It means you're putting off the side effects of surgery or radiation therapy. Having surgery or radiation therapy is no guarantee that a man will live longer than a man who chooses to put off treatment.

If you and your doctor agree that active surveillance is a good idea, your doctor will check you regularly (such as every 3 to 6 months, at first). After about one year, your doctor may order another biopsy to check the Gleason score. You may begin treatment if your Gleason score rises, your PSA level starts to rise, or you develop symptoms. You'll receive surgery, radiation therapy, or another approach.

Active surveillance avoids or delays the side effects of surgery and radiation therapy, but this choice has risks. For some men, it may reduce the chance to control cancer before it spreads. Also, it may be harder to cope with surgery or radiation therapy when you're older.

If you choose active surveillance but grow concerned later, you should discuss your feelings with your doctor. Another approach is an option for most men.

questions before choosing active surveillance:

- If I choose active surveillance, can I change my mind later on?
- Is it safe for me to put off treatment?
- How often will I have checkups? Which tests will I need? Will I need a repeat biopsy?
- How will we know if the prostate cancer is getting worse?
- Between checkups, what problems should I tell you about?

Surgery

Surgery is an option for men with early (Stage I or II) prostate cancer. It's sometimes an option for men with Stage III or IV prostate cancer. The surgeon may remove the whole prostate or only part of it.

Before the surgeon removes the prostate, the lymph nodes in the pelvis may be removed. If prostate cancer cells are found in the lymph nodes, the disease may have spread to other parts of the body. If cancer has spread to the lymph nodes, the surgeon does not always remove the prostate and may suggest other types of treatment.

There are several types of surgery for prostate cancer. Each type has benefits and risks. You and your doctor can talk about the types of surgery and which may be right for you:

• Open surgery: The surgeon makes a large incision (cut) into your body to remove the tumor. There are two approaches:

— Through the abdomen: The surgeon removes the entire prostate through a cut in the abdomen. This is called a radical retropubic prostatectomy.

— Between the scrotum and anus: The surgeon removes the entire prostate through a cut between the scrotum and the anus. This is called a radical perineal prostatectomy.

• Laparoscopic prostatectomy: The surgeon removes the entire prostate through small cuts, rather than a single long cut in the abdomen. A thin, lighted tube (a laparoscope) helps the surgeon remove the prostate.

• Robotic laparoscopic surgery: The surgeon removes the entire prostate through small cuts. A laparoscope and a robot are used to help remove the prostate. The surgeon uses handles below a computer display to control the robot's arms.

• Cryosurgery: For some men, cryosurgery is an option. The surgeon inserts a tool through a small cut between the scrotum and anus. The tool freezes and kills prostate tissue. Cryosurgery is under study. See the section on Taking Part in Cancer Research on page 32.

• TURP: A man with advanced prostate cancer may choose TURP (transurethral resection of the prostate) to relieve symptoms. The surgeon inserts a long, thin scope through the urethra. A cutting tool at the end of the scope removes tissue from the inside of the prostate. TURP may not remove all of the cancer, but it can remove tissue that blocks the flow of urine.

You may be uncomfortable for the first few days or weeks after surgery. However, medicine can help control the pain. Before surgery, you should discuss the plan for pain relief with your doctor or nurse. After surgery, your doctor can adjust the plan if you need more pain relief.

The time it takes to heal after surgery is different for each man and depends on the type of surgery. You may be in the hospital for one to three days.

After surgery, the urethra needs time to heal. You'll have a catheter. A catheter is a tube put through the urethra into the bladder to drain urine. You'll have the catheter for 5 days to 3 weeks. Your nurse or doctor will show you how to care for it.

After surgery, some men may lose control of the flow of urine (urinary incontinence). Most men regain at least some bladder control after a few weeks.

Surgery can damage the nerves around the prostate. Damaging these nerves can make a man impotent (unable to have an erection). In some cases, your surgeon can protect the nerves that control erection. But if you have a large tumor or a tumor that's very close to the nerves, surgery may cause impotence. Impotence can be permanent. You can talk with your doctor about medicine and other ways to help manage the sexual side effects of cancer treatment.

If your prostate is removed, you will no longer produce semen. You'll have dry orgasms. If you wish to father children, you may consider sperm banking or a sperm retrieval procedure before surgery.

You may want to ask your doctor these questions before choosing surgery:

- What kinds of surgery can I consider? Which operation do you recommend for me? Why?
- How long will I be in the hospital after surgery?
- How will I feel after the operation?
- If I have pain, how can we control it?

- Will I have any lasting side effects? What is the chance that the surgery will cause incontinence or impotence?

- Is there someone that I can talk with who has had the same surgery that I'll be having?
- How often will I need checkups?

Radiation Therapy

Radiation therapy is an option for men with any stage of prostate cancer. Men with early stage prostate cancer may choose radiation therapy instead of surgery. It also may be used after surgery to destroy any cancer cells that remain in the area.

In later stages of prostate cancer, radiation treatment may be used to help relieve pain.

Radiation therapy (also called radiotherapy) uses high-energy rays to kill cancer cells. It affects cells only in the treated area.

Doctors use two types of radiation therapy to treat prostate cancer. Some men receive both types:

• External radiation: The radiation comes from a large machine outside the body. You will go to a hospital or clinic for treatment. Treatments are usually 5 days a week for several weeks. Many men receive 3-dimensional conformal radiation therapy or intensity-modulated radiation therapy. These types of treatment use computers to more closely target the cancer to lessen the damage to healthy tissue near the prostate.

• Internal radiation (implant radiation or brachytherapy): The radiation comes from radioactive material usually contained in very small implants called seeds. Dozens of seeds are placed inside needles, and the needles are inserted into the prostate. The needles are removed, leaving the seeds behind. The seeds give off radiation for months. They don't need to be removed once the radiation is gone.

Side effects depend mainly on the dose and type of radiation. You're likely to be very tired during radiation therapy, especially in the later weeks of treatment. Resting is important, but doctors usually advise patients to try to stay active, unless it leads to pain or other problems.

If you have external radiation, you may have diarrhea or frequent and uncomfortable urination. Some men have lasting bowel or urinary problems. Your skin in the treated area may become red, dry, and tender. You may lose hair in the treated area. The hair may not grow back.

Internal radiation therapy may cause incontinence. This side effect usually goes away.

Both internal and external radiation can cause impotence. You can talk with your doctor about ways to help cope with this side effect.

You may find it helpful to read the NCI booklet Radiation Therapy and You.

You may want to ask your doctor these questions before choosing radiation therapy:

• Which type of radiation therapy can I consider? Are both types an option for me?

• When will treatment start? When will it end? How often will I have treatments?

• Will I need to stay in the hospital?

• What can I do to take care of myself before, during, and after treatment?

- How will I feel during treatment? Will I be able to drive myself to and from treatment?
- How will we know the treatment is working?
- How will I feel after the radiation therapy?
- Are there any lasting effects?

- What is the chance that the cancer will come back in my prostate?
- How often will I need checkups?

Hormone Therapy

A man with prostate cancer may have hormone therapy before, during, or after radiation therapy. Hormone therapy is also used alone for prostate cancer that has returned after treatment.

Male hormones (androgens) can cause prostate cancer to grow. Hormone therapy keeps prostate cancer cells from getting the male hormones they need to grow. The testicles are the body's main source of the male hormone testosterone. The adrenal gland makes other male hormones and a small amount of

testosterone.

Hormone therapy uses drugs or surgery:

- Drugs: Your doctor may suggest a drug that can block natural hormones:

— Luteinizing hormone-releasing hormone (LH-RH) agonists: These drugs can prevent the testicles from making testosterone. Examples are leuprolide, goserelin, and triptorelin. The testosterone level falls slowly. Without

testosterone, the tumor shrinks, or its growth slows. These drugs are also called gonadotropinreleasing hormone (GnRH) agonists.

— Antiandrogens: These drugs can block the action of male hormones. Examples are flutamide, bicalutamide, and nilutamide.

— Other drugs: Some drugs can prevent the adrenal gland from making testosterone. Examples are ketoconazole and

aminoglutethimide.

- Surgery: Surgery to remove the testicles is called orchiectomy.

After orchiectomy or treatment with an LH-RH agonist, your body no longer gets testosterone from the testicles, the major source of male hormones. Because the adrenal gland makes small amounts of male hormones, you may receive an antiandrogen to block the action of the male hormones that remain. This combination of treatments is known as total androgen blockade (also called combined androgen blockade). However, studies have shown that total androgen blockade is no more effective than surgery or an LH-RH agonist alone.

Hormone therapy causes side effects such as impotence, hot flashes, and loss of sexual desire. Also, any treatment that lowers hormone levels can weaken your bones. Your doctor can suggest medicines that may reduce your risk of bone fractures.

An LH-RH agonist may make your symptoms worse for a short time at first. This temporary problem is called "flare." To prevent flare, your doctor may give you an antiandrogen for a few weeks along with the LH-RH agonist.

An LH-RH agonist such as leuprolide can increase body fat, especially around the waist. The levels of sugar and cholesterol in your blood may increase too. Because these changes increase the risk of diabetes and heart disease, your health care team will monitor you for these side effects.

Antiandrogens (such as nilutamide) can cause nausea, diarrhea, or breast growth or tenderness. Rarely, they may cause liver problems (pain in the abdomen, yellow eyes, or dark urine). Some men who use nilutamide may have shortness of breath or develop heart failure. Some may have trouble adjusting to sudden changes in light.

If you receive total androgen blockade, you may have more side effects than if you have just one type of hormone treatment.

If used for a long time, ketoconazole may cause liver problems, and aminoglutethimide can cause skin rashes.

Doctors usually treat prostate cancer that has spread to other parts of the body with hormone therapy. For some men, the cancer will be controlled for two or three years, but others will have a much shorter response to hormone therapy. In time, most prostate cancers can grow with very little or no male hormones, and hormone therapy alone is no longer helpful. At that time, your doctor may suggest chemotherapy or other forms of treatment that are under study. In many cases, the doctor may suggest continuing with hormone therapy because it may still be effective against some of the cancer cells.

You may want to ask your doctor these questions before choosing hormone therapy:
• Which kind of hormone therapy can I consider? Would you recommend drugs or surgery? Why?

• If I have drugs, when will treatment start? How often will I have treatments? When will treatment end?

- If I have surgery, how long will I need to stay in the hospital?
- How will I feel during treatment?
- What can I do to take care of myself during treatment?
- How will we know the treatment is working?
- Which side effects should I tell you about?
- Will there be lasting side effects?
- How often will I need checkups?

Chemotherapy

Chemotherapy may be used for prostate cancer that has spread and no longer responds to hormone therapy.

Chemotherapy uses drugs to kill cancer cells. The drugs for prostate cancer are usually given through a vein (intravenous). You may receive chemotherapy in a clinic, at the doctor's office, or at home. Some men need to stay in the hospital during treatment.

The side effects depend mainly on which drugs are given and how much. Chemotherapy kills fast-growing cancer cells, but the drugs can also harm normal cells that divide rapidly:

• Blood cells: When chemotherapy lowers the levels of healthy blood cells, you're more likely to get infections, bruise or bleed easily, and feel very weak and tired. Your health care team will check for low levels of blood cells. If your levels are low, your health care team may stop the chemotherapy for a while or reduce the dose of drug. There are also medicines that can help your body make new blood cells.

• Cells in hair roots: Chemotherapy may cause hair loss. If you lose your hair, it will grow back, but it may change in color and texture.

• Cells that line the digestive tract: Chemotherapy can cause a poor appetite, nausea and vomiting, or diarrhea. Your health care team can give you medicines and suggest other ways to help with these problems.

Other side effects include shortness of breath and a problem with your body holding extra water. Your health care team can give you medicine to protect against too much water building up in the body. Also, chemotherapy may cause a skin rash, tingling or numbness in your hands and feet, and watery eyes. Your health care team can suggest ways to control many of these problems. Most go away when treatment ends.

You may wish to read the NCI booklet Chemotherapy and You.

You may want to ask your doctor these questions before choosing chemotherapy:

• Why do I need this treatment?

- Which drug or drugs will I have?
- How do the drugs work?

- What are the expected benefits of the treatment?
- What are the risks and possible side effects of treatment? What can we do about them?
- When will treatment start? When will it end?
- How will treatment affect my normal activities?

Second Opinion

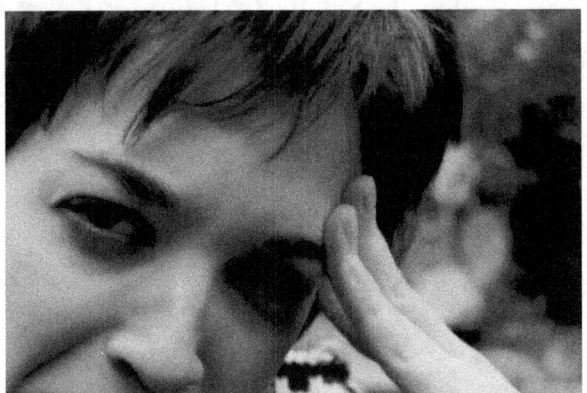

Before starting treatment, you might want a second opinion about your diagnosis and treatment plan. You may even want to talk to several different doctors about all of the treatment options, their side effects, and the expected results. For example, you may want to talk to a urologist, radiation oncologist, and medical oncologist.

Some people worry that the doctor will be offended if they ask for a second opinion. Usually the opposite is true. Most doctors welcome a second opinion. And many health insurance companies will pay for a second opinion if you or your doctor requests it.

If you get a second opinion, the doctor may agree with your first doctor's diagnosis and treatment plan. Or, the second doctor may suggest another approach. Either way, you have more information and perhaps a greater sense of control. You can feel more confident about the decisions you make, knowing that you've looked at your options.

It may take some time and effort to gather your medical records and see another doctor. In most cases, it's not a problem to take several weeks to get a second opinion. The delay in starting treatment usually will not make treatment less effective. To make sure, you should discuss this delay with your doctor.

There are many ways to find a doctor for a second opinion. You can ask your doctor, a local or state medical society, a nearby hospital, or a medical school for names of specialists. NCI's Cancer Information Service at 1–800–4–CANCER can tell you about nearby treatment centers. Other sources can be found in the NCI fact sheet How To Find a Doctor or Treatment Facility If You Have Cancer.

Nutrition and Physical Activity

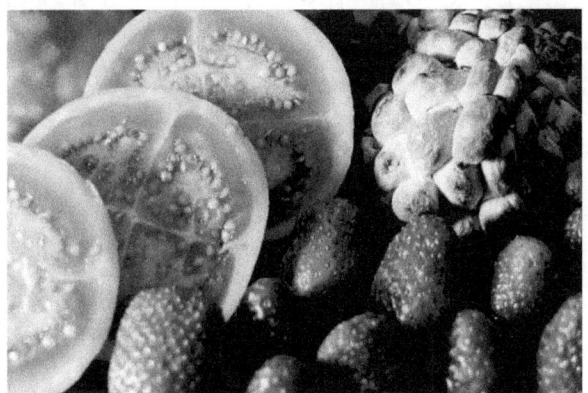

It's important for you to take care of yourself by eating well and staying as active as you can.

You need the right amount of calories to maintain a good weight. You also need enough protein to keep up your strength. Eating well may help you feel better and have more energy.

Your doctor, a registered dietitian, or another health care provider can suggest a healthy diet. Also, the NCI booklet Eating Hints for Cancer Patients has many useful ideas and recipes.

Research shows that people with cancer feel better when they are active. Walking, yoga, swimming, and other activities can increase your energy. Exercise may reduce pain and make treatment easier to handle. It also can help relieve stress. Whatever physical activity you choose, be sure to talk to your doctor before you start. Also, if your activity causes you pain or other problems, be sure to let your doctor or nurse know about it. You shouldn't try to exercise to the point of exhaustion

Follow-up Care

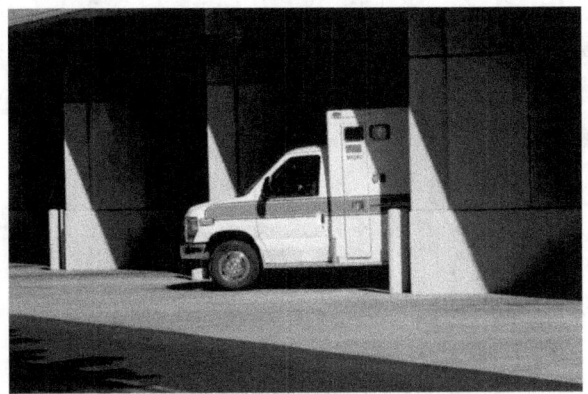

You'll need regular checkups after treatment for prostate cancer. Checkups help ensure that any changes in your health are noted and treated if needed. If you have any health problems between checkups, you should contact your doctor.

Your doctor will check for return of cancer. Even when the cancer seems to have been completely removed or destroyed, the disease sometimes returns because undetected cancer cells remained somewhere in the body after treatment.

Checkups may include a digital rectal exam and a PSA test. A rise in PSA level can mean that cancer has returned after treatment. Your doctor may also order a biopsy, a bone scan, CT scans, an MRI, or other tests.

The NCI has publications to help answer questions about follow-up care and other concerns. You may find it helpful to read the NCI booklet Facing Forward: Life After Cancer Treatment. You may also want to read the NCI fact sheet Follow-up Care After Cancer Treatment: Questions and Answers.

You may want to ask your doctor these questions after you have finished treatment:

- How often will I need checkups?
- Which follow-up tests do you suggest for me?

- Between checkups, what health problems or symptoms should I tell you about?

Sources of Support

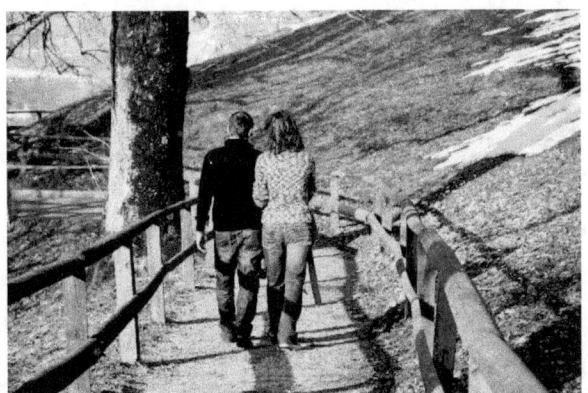

Learning you have prostate cancer can change your life and the lives of those close to you. These changes can be hard to handle. It's normal for you, your family, and your friends to need help coping with the feelings that a diagnosis of cancer can bring.

Concerns about treatments and managing side effects, hospital stays, and medical bills are common. You may also worry about caring for your family, keeping your job, or continuing daily activities.

Here's where you can go for support:

• Doctors, nurses, and other members of your health care team can answer questions about treatment, working, or other activities.

• Social workers, counselors, or members of the clergy can be helpful if you want to talk about your feelings or concerns. Often, social workers can suggest resources for financial aid, transportation, home care, or emotional support.

• Support groups also can help. In these groups, patients or their family members meet with other patients or their families to share what they have learned about coping with the disease and the effects of treatment. Groups may offer support in person, over the telephone, or on the Internet. You may want to talk with a member of your health care team about finding a support group.

• Information specialists at 1–800–4–CANCER and at LiveHelp (http://www.cancer.gov/help) can help you locate programs, services, and publications. They can send you a list of organizations that offer services to people with cancer.

• Your doctor or a sex counselor may be helpful if you and your partner are concerned about the effects of prostate cancer on your sexual relationship. Ask your doctor about possible treatment of side effects and whether these effects are likely to last. Whatever the outlook, you and your partner may find it helps to discuss your concerns.

For tips on coping, you may want to read the NCI booklet Taking Time: Support for People With Cancer.

Taking Part in Cancer Research

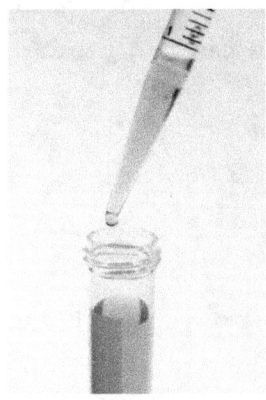

Cancer research has led to real progress in prostate cancer detection, treatment, and supportive care. Because of research, men with prostate cancer can look forward to a better quality of life and less chance of dying from the disease. Continuing research offers hope that, in the future, even more men with this disease will be treated successfully.

Doctors all over the country are conducting many types of clinical trials (research studies in which people volunteer to take part). Clinical trials are designed to answer important questions and to find out whether new approaches are safe and effective.

Doctors are studying many types of treatment and their combinations:

• Active surveillance: Doctors are comparing having surgery or radiation right away to choosing active surveillance. The results of the study will help doctors know whether to treat early stage prostate cancer right away, or only when symptoms appear or get worse.

• Cryosurgery: Surgeons are studying a tool that freezes and kills prostate tissue in men with early prostate cancer.

• High-intensity focused ultrasound (HIFU): Doctors are testing HIFU in men with early prostate cancer. A probe is placed in the rectum. The probe gives off high-intensity ultrasound waves that heat up and destroy the prostate tumor.

• Radiation therapy: Doctors are using different doses or schedules of radiation therapy. They are looking at the use of radioactive implants after external radiation. And they are combining radiation therapy with other treatments, such as hormone therapy.

• Hormone therapy: Researchers are studying different schedules of hormone therapy, and they are combining it with other treatments.

• Chemotherapy: Researchers are testing anticancer drugs and combining them with hormone therapy or biological therapy. Chemotherapy allows some men to live longer and with a better quality of life.

•   Biological therapy: New biological therapies are under study. For example, doctors are testing cancer vaccines that help the immune system kill cancer cells.

Doctors are also testing ways to manage the problems caused by prostate cancer and its treatment. For example, they are studying ways to manage or prevent bone pain, bone thinning, hot flashes, and impotence.

Even if the men in a trial do not benefit directly, they may still make an important contribution by helping doctors learn more about prostate cancer and how to control it. Although clinical trials may pose some risks, doctors do all they can to protect their patients.

If you're interested in being part of a clinical trial, talk with your doctor. You may want to read the NCI booklet Taking Part in Cancer Treatment Research Studies. It describes how treatment studies are carried out and explains their possible benefits and risks.

NCI's Web site includes a section on clinical trials at http://www.cancer.gov/clinicaltrials. It has general information about clinical trials as well as detailed information about specific

ongoing studies of prostate cancer. NCI's Information Specialists at 1–800–4–CANCER or at LiveHelp at

http://www.cancer.gov/help can answer questions and
provide information about clinical trials.

Dictionary

Definitions of thousands of terms are on the NCI Web site in the NCI Dictionary of Cancer Terms. You can access it at http://www.cancer.gov/dictionary.

3-dimensional conformal radiation therapy (3-dihMEN-shuh-nul kun-FOR-mul RAY-dee-AY-shun THAYR-uh-pee): A procedure that uses a computer to create a 3-dimensional picture of the tumor. This allows doctors to give the highest possible dose of radiation to the tumor, while sparing the normal tissue as much as possible.

Abdomen (AB-doh-men): The area of the body that contains the pancreas, stomach, intestines, liver, gallbladder, and other organs.

Active surveillance (ser-VAY-lents): Closely monitoring a patient's condition but withholding treatment until symptoms appear or change. Also called observation, watchful waiting, or expectant management.

Adrenal gland (uh-DREE-nul): A small gland that makes steroid hormones, adrenaline, and noradrenaline. These hormones help control heart rate, blood pressure, and other important body functions. There are two adrenal glands, one on top of each kidney. Also called suprarenal gland.

Aminoglutethimide (a-MEE-no-gloo-TETH-ih-mide): An anticancer drug that belongs to the family of drugs called nonsteroidal aromatase inhibitors. It is used to decrease the production of sex hormones (estrogen in women or testosterone in men) and suppress the growth of tumors that need sex hormones to grow.

Androgen (AN-droh-jen): A type of hormone that promotes the development and maintenance of male sex characteristics.

Antiandrogen (AN-tee-AN-droh-jen): A substance that prevents cells from making or using androgens (hormones that play a role in the formation of male sex characteristics).

Anus (AY-nus): The opening of the rectum to the outside of the body.

Benign (beh-NINE): Not cancerous. Benign tumors may grow larger but do not spread to other parts of the body.

Benign prostatic hyperplasia (beh-NINE prah-STA-tik HY-per-PLAY-zhuh): BPH. A benign (noncancerous) condition in which an overgrowth of prostate tissue pushes against the urethra and the bladder, blocking the flow of urine. Also called benign prostatic hypertrophy.

Bicalutamide (bye-ka-LOO-ta-mide): An anticancer drug that belongs to the family of drugs called antiandrogens.

Biological therapy (BY-oh-LAH-jih-kul THAYR-uhpee): Treatment to boost or restore the ability of the immune system to fight cancer, infections, and other diseases. Also used to lessen certain side effects that may be caused by some cancer treatments. Also called immunotherapy, biotherapy, biological response modifier therapy, and BRM therapy.

Biopsy (BY-op-see): The removal of cells or tissues for examination by a pathologist. The pathologist may study the tissue under a microscope or perform other tests on the cells or tissue. There are many different types of biopsy procedures. The most common types include: (1) incisional biopsy, in which only a sample of tissue is removed; (2) excisional biopsy, in which an entire lump or suspicious area is removed; and (3) needle biopsy, in which a sample of tissue or fluid is removed with a needle. When a wide needle is used, the procedure is called a core biopsy. When a thin needle is used, the procedure is called a fine-needle aspiration biopsy.

Bladder (BLA-der): The organ that stores urine.

Bone scan : A technique to create images of bones on a computer screen or on film. A small amount of radioactive material is injected into a blood vessel and travels through the bloodstream; it collects in the bones and is detected by a scanner.

Brachytherapy (BRAY-kee-THAYR-uh-pee): A type of radiation therapy in which radioactive material sealed in needles, seeds, wires, or catheters is placed directly into or near a tumor. Also called radiation
brachytherapy, internal radiation therapy, and implant radiation therapy.

BRCA1 : A gene on chromosome 17 that normally helps to suppress cell growth. A person who inherits a mutated (changed) BRCA1 gene has a higher risk of getting breast, ovarian, or prostate cancer.

BRCA2 : A gene on chromosome 13 that normally helps to suppress cell growth. A person who inherits a mutated (changed) BRCA2 gene has a higher risk of getting breast, ovarian, or prostate cancer.

Cancer (KAN-ser): A term for diseases in which abnormal cells divide without control. Cancer cells can invade nearby tissues and can spread to other parts of the body through the blood and lymph systems.

Catheter (KA-theh-ter): A flexible tube used to deliver fluids into or withdraw fluids from the body.

Cell : The individual unit that makes up the tissues of the body. All living things are made up of one or more cells.

Chemotherapy (KEE-moh-THAYR-uh-pee): Treatment with drugs that kill cancer cells.

Cholesterol (kuh-LESS-tuh-rawl): A waxy, fat-like substance made in the liver and found in the blood and in all cells of the body. Cholesterol also comes from eating foods taken from animals such as egg yolks, meat, and whole-milk dairy products.

Chromosome (KROH-muh-some): Part of a cell that contains genetic information. Except for sperm and eggs, all human cells contain 46 chromosomes.

Clinical trial : A type of research study that tests how well new medical approaches work in people. These studies test new methods of screening, prevention, diagnosis, or treatment of a disease.

Contrast material : A dye or other substance that helps to show abnormal areas inside the body. It is given by injection into a vein, by enema, or by mouth. Contrast material may be used with x-rays, CT scans, MRI, or other imaging tests.

Cryosurgery (KRY-oh-SER-juh-ree): A procedure in which tissue is frozen to destroy abnormal cells. This is usually done with a special instrument that contains liquid nitrogen or liquid carbon dioxide. Also called cryoablation.

CT scan : Computed tomography scan (kum-PYOO-ted tuh-MAH-gruh-fee skan). A series of detailed pictures of areas inside the body taken from different angles; the pictures are created by a computer linked to an x-ray machine. Also called computerized tomography and computerized axial tomography (CAT) scan.

Digestive tract (dy-JES-tiv): The organs through which food and liquids pass when they are swallowed, digested, and eliminated. These organs are the mouth, esophagus, stomach, small and large intestines, and rectum.

Digital rectal examination (DIH-jih-tul REK-tul eg-zam-ih-NAY-shun): DRE. An examination in which a doctor inserts a lubricated, gloved finger into the rectum to feel for abnormalities.

Dry orgasm: Sexual climax without the release of semen from the penis.

Ejaculation (i-JAK-yoo-LAY-shun): The release of semen through the penis during orgasm.

Erection (ih-REK-shun): In medicine, the swelling of the penis with blood, causing it to become firm.

External radiation therapy (RAY-dee-AY-shun THAYR-uh-pee): A type of radiation therapy that uses a machine to aim high-energy rays at the cancer from outside of the body. Also called external beam radiation therapy.

Flutamide (FLOO-ta-mide): An anticancer drug that is a type of antiandrogen.

Gene : The functional and physical unit of heredity passed from parent to offspring. Genes are pieces of DNA, and most genes contain the information for making a specific protein.

Genome: The complete genetic material of an organism.

Gland : An organ that makes one or more substances, such as hormones, digestive juices, sweat, tears, saliva, or milk.

Gleason score (GLEE-sun): A system of grading prostate cancer tissue based on how it looks under a microscope. Gleason scores range from 2 to 10 and indicate how likely it is that a tumor will spread. A low Gleason score means the cancer tissue is similar to normal prostate tissue and the tumor is less likely to spread; a high Gleason score means the cancer tissue is very different from normal and the tumor is more likely to spread.

Gonadotropin-releasing hormone agonist : A hormone made in the laboratory that has the same effect as the gonadotropin-releasing hormone (GnRH) produced naturally by the body.

Goserelin (go-SAIR-uh-lin): A drug that belongs to the family of drugs called gonadotropin-releasing hormone analogs. Goserelin is used to block hormone production in the ovaries or testicles.

Grade: The grade of a tumor depends on how abnormal the cancer cells look under a microscope and how quickly the tumor is likely to grow and spread. Grading systems are different for each type of cancer.

Green tea extract : A substance that is being studied in the prevention of cancer. It is made from decaffeinated green tea, and contains chemicals called catechins, which are antioxidants. Also called Polyphenon E. High-intensity focused ultrasound (UL-truhSOWND): HIFU. A type of therapy that is being studied for certain cancers. A probe gives off highintensity ultrasound waves that heat up and destroy the tumor.

Hormone (HOR-mone): One of many chemicals made by glands in the body. Hormones circulate in the bloodstream and control the actions of certain cells or organs. Some hormones can also be made in the laboratory.

Hormone therapy (HOR-mone THAYR-uh-pee): Treatment that adds, blocks, or removes hormones. For certain conditions (such as diabetes or menopause), hormones are given to adjust low hormone levels. To slow or stop the growth of certain cancers (such as prostate or breast cancer), synthetic hormones or other drugs may be given to block the body's natural hormones. Sometimes surgery is needed to remove the gland that makes a certain hormone. Also called hormonal therapy, hormone treatment, or endocrine therapy.

Immune system (ih-MYOON): The complex group of organs and cells that defends the body against infections and other diseases.

Implant radiation therapy (RAY-dee-AY-shun THAYR-uh-pee): A type of radiation therapy in which radioactive material sealed in needles, seeds, wires, or catheters is placed directly into or near a tumor. Also called brachytherapy, radiation brachytherapy, and internal radiation therapy.

Impotent (IM-po-tent): In medicine, describes the inability to have an erection of the penis adequate for sexual intercourse.

Incision (in-SIH-zhun): A cut made in the body to perform surgery.

Incontinence (in-KAHN-tih-nens): Inability to control the flow of urine from the bladder (urinary incontinence) or the escape of stool from the rectum (fecal incontinence).

Inflammation (IN-fluh-MAY-shun): Redness, swelling, pain, and/or a feeling of heat in an area of the body. This is a protective reaction to injury, disease, or irritation of the tissues.

Injection: Use of a syringe and needle to push fluids or drugs into the body; often called a "shot."

Intensity-modulated radiation therapy (in-TEN-sihtee-MAH-juh-LAY-tid RAY-dee-AY-shun THAYR-uhpee): A type of 3-dimensional radiation therapy that uses computer-generated images to show the size and shape of the tumor. Thin beams of radiation of different intensities are aimed at the tumor from many angles. This type of radiation therapy reduces the damage to healthy tissue near the tumor.

Internal radiation therapy (in-TER-nul RAY-dee-AYshun THAYR-uh-pee): A type of radiation therapy in which radioactive material sealed in needles, seeds, wires, or catheters is placed directly into or near a tumor. Also called brachytherapy, radiation

brachytherapy, and implant radiation therapy.

Intravenous (IN-truh-VEE-nus): IV. Into or within a vein. Intravenous usually refers to a way of giving a drug or other substance through a needle or tube inserted into a vein.

Ketoconazole (kee-ta-KOE-na-zol): A drug that treats infection caused by a fungus. It is also used as a treatment for prostate cancer because it can block the production of male sex hormones.

Laparoscope (LA-puh-ruh-SKOPE): A thin, tube-like instrument used to look at tissues and organs inside the abdomen. A laparoscope has a light and a lens for viewing and may have a tool to remove tissue. Laparoscopic prostatectomy (LA-puh-ruh-SKAH-pik PROS-tuh-TEK-toh-mee): Surgery to remove all or part of the prostate with the aid of a laparoscope. A laparoscope is a thin, tube-like instrument with a light and a lens for viewing. It may also have a tool to remove tissue.

Leuprolide (LOO-pro-lide): A drug used to treat symptoms of advanced prostate cancer. It is also used to treat early puberty in children and certain

gynecologic conditions. It is being studied in the treatment of other conditions and types of cancer. Leuprolide blocks the body from making testosterone (a male hormone) and estradiol (a female hormone). It may stop the growth of prostate cancer cells that need testosterone to grow. It is a type of gonadotropinreleasing hormone analog.

Local anesthesia (A-nes-THEE-zhuh): Drugs that cause a temporary loss of feeling in one part of the body. The patient remains awake but has no feeling in the part of the body treated with the anesthetic. Luteinizing hormone-releasing hormone agonist (LOO-tin-eye-zing. . .AG-o-nist): LH-RH agonist. A drug that inhibits the secretion of sex hormones. In men, LH-RH agonist causes testosterone levels to fall. In women, LH-RH agonist causes the levels of estrogen and other sex hormones to fall.

Lymph node (limf node): A rounded mass of lymphatic tissue that is surrounded by a capsule of connective tissue. Lymph nodes filter lymph (lymphatic fluid), and they store lymphocytes (white blood cells). They are located along lymphatic vessels. Also called a lymph gland.

Lymph vessel (limf): A thin tube that carries lymph (lymphatic fluid) and white blood cells through the lymphatic system. Also called lymphatic vessel.

Malignant (muh-LIG-nunt): Cancerous. Malignant tumors can invade and destroy nearby tissue and spread to other parts of the body.

Medical oncologist (MEH-dih-kul on-KAH-loh-jist): A doctor who specializes in diagnosing and treating cancer using chemotherapy, hormonal therapy, and biological therapy. A medical oncologist often is the main health care provider for someone who has cancer. A medical oncologist also gives supportive care and may coordinate treatment given by other specialists.

Metastasis (meh-TAS-tuh-sis): The spread of cancer from one part of the body to another. A tumor formed by cells that have spread is called a "metastatic tumor" or a "metastasis." The metastatic tumor contains cells that are like those in the original (primary) tumor. The plural form of metastasis is metastases (meh-TAS-tuhseez).

MRI : Magnetic resonance imaging (mag-NEH-tik REH-zuh-nunts IH-muh-jing). A procedure in which radio waves and a powerful magnet linked to a computer are used to create detailed pictures of areas inside the body.

Nerve: A bundle of fibers that receives and sends messages between the body and the brain. The messages are sent by chemical and electrical changes in the cells that make up the nerves.

Nilutamide (ny-LOO-tuh-mide): A drug that blocks the effects of male hormones in the body. It is a type of antiandrogen.

Oncology nurse (on-KAH-loh-jee): A nurse who specializes in caring for people who have cancer.

Orchiectomy (or-kee-EK-toh-mee): Surgery to remove one or both testicles. Also called orchidectomy. Organ: A part of the body that performs a specific function. For example, the heart is an organ.

Pathologist (puh-THAH-loh-jist): A doctor who identifies diseases by studying cells and tissues under a microscope.

Pelvis: The lower part of the abdomen, located between the hip bones.

Penis : An external male reproductive organ. It contains a tube called the urethra, which carries semen and urine to the outside of the body.

Prostate (PROS-tayt): A gland in the male reproductive system. The prostate surrounds the part of the urethra (the tube that empties the bladder) just below the bladder, and produces a fluid that forms part of the semen.

Prostate-specific antigen (PROS-tayt-speh-SIH-fik AN-tih-jen): PSA. A substance produced by the prostate that may be found in an increased amount in the blood of men who have prostate cancer, benign prostatic hyperplasia, or infection or inflammation of the prostate.

Prostatic intraepithelial neoplasia (prah-STA-tik IN-truh-eh-puh-THEE-lee-ul NEE-oh-PLAY-zhuh): PIN. Non-cancerous growth of the cells lining the internal and external surfaces of the prostate gland. Having high-grade PIN may increase the risk of developing prostate cancer.

Prostatitis (prah-stuh-TY-tis): Inflammation of the prostate gland.

Radiation (RAY-dee-AY-shun): Energy released in the form of particles or electromagnetic waves. Common sources of radiation include radon gas, cosmic rays from outer space, and medical x-rays.

Radiation oncologist (RAY-dee-AY-shun on-KAH-lohjist): A doctor who specializes in using radiation to treat cancer.

Radiation therapy (RAY-dee-AY-shun THAYR-uhpee): The use of high-energy radiation from x-rays, gamma rays, neutrons, and other sources to kill cancer cells and shrink tumors. Radiation may come from a machine outside the body (external beam radiation therapy), or it may come from radioactive material placed in the body near cancer cells (internal radiation therapy). Systemic radiation therapy uses a radioactive substance, such as a radiolabeled monoclonal antibody, that travels in the blood to tissues throughout the body. Also called radiotherapy and irradiation.

Radical perineal prostatectomy (RA-dih-kul PAYR-ihNEE-ul PROS-tuh-TEK-toh-mee): Surgery to remove all of the prostate through an incision between the scrotum and the anus. Nearby lymph nodes are sometimes removed through a separate incision in the wall of the abdomen.

Radical retropubic prostatectomy (RA-dih-kul reh-troh-PYOO-bik PROS-tuh-TEK-toh-mee): Surgery to remove all of the prostate and nearby lymph nodes through an incision in the wall of the abdomen. Radioactive (RAY-dee-oh-AK-tiv): Giving off radiation.

Rectum : The last several inches of the large intestine. The rectum ends at the anus.

Registered dietitian (dy-eh-TIH-shun): A health professional with special training in the use of diet and nutrition to keep the body healthy. A registered dietitian may help the medical team improve the nutritional health of a patient.

Reproductive system (REE-pruh-DUK-tiv): The organs involved in producing offspring. In women, this system includes the ovaries, the fallopian tubes, the uterus (womb), the cervix, and the vagina (birth canal). In men, it includes the prostate, the testes, and the penis.

Risk factor : Something that may increase the chance of developing a disease. Some examples of risk factors for cancer include age, a family history of certain cancers, use of tobacco products, certain eating habits, obesity, lack of exercise, exposure to radiation or other cancer-causing agents, and certain genetic changes.

Scrotum (SKRO-tum): In males, the external sac that contains the testicles.

Selenium (suh-LEE-nee-um): A mineral that is needed by the body to stay healthy. It is being studied in the prevention and treatment of some types of cancer. Selenium is a type of antioxidant.

Semen : The fluid that is released through the penis during orgasm. Semen is made up of sperm from the testicles and fluid from the prostate and other sex glands.

Seminal fluid (SEM-in-al): Fluid from the prostate and other sex glands that helps transport sperm out of the man's body during orgasm.

Seminal vesicle (SEM-in-al VES-ih-kul): A gland that helps produce semen.

Side effect : A problem that occurs when treatment affects healthy tissues or organs. Some common side effects of cancer treatment are fatigue, pain, nausea, vomiting, decreased blood cell counts, hair loss, and mouth sores.

Sonogram (SON-o-gram): A computer picture of areas inside the body created by bouncing high-energy sound waves (ultrasound) off internal tissues or organs. Also called an ultrasonogram.

Sperm: The male reproductive cell, formed in the testicle. A sperm unites with an egg to form an embryo.

Sperm banking : Freezing sperm for use in the future. This procedure can allow men to father children after loss of fertility.

Sperm retrieval (rih-TREE-vul): Removal of sperm from a man's testis or epididymis by a doctor using a fine needle or another instrument.

Supportive care : Care given to improve the quality of life of patients who have a serious or life-threatening disease. The goal of supportive care is to prevent or treat as early as possible the symptoms of the disease, side effects caused by treatment of the disease, and psychological, social, and spiritual problems related to the disease or its treatment. Also called palliative care, comfort care, and symptom management.

Surgeon: A doctor who removes or repairs a part of the body by operating on the patient.

Surgery (SER-juh-ree): A procedure to remove or repair a part of the body or to find out whether disease is present. An operation.

Testicle (TES-tih-kul): One of two egg-shaped glands found inside the scrotum that produce sperm and male hormones. Also called a testis.

Testosterone (tes-TOS-ter-own): A hormone that promotes the development and maintenance of male sex characteristics.

Tissue (TISH-oo): A group or layer of cells that work together to perform a specific function.

Total androgen blockade (AN-droh-jen): Therapy used to eliminate male sex hormones (androgens) in the body. This may be done with surgery, hormonal therapy, or a combination.

Transrectal biopsy (TRANZ-REK-tul BY-op-see): A procedure in which a sample of tissue is removed from the prostate using a thin needle that is inserted through the rectum and into the prostate. Transrectal ultrasound (TRUS) is usually used to guide the needle. The sample is examined under a microscope to see if it contains cancer.

Transrectal ultrasound (TRANZ-REK-tul UL-truhSOWND): TRUS. A procedure in which a probe that sends out high-energy sound waves is inserted into the rectum. The sound waves are bounced off internal tissues or organs and make echoes. The echoes form a picture of body tissue called a sonogram. TRUS is used to look for abnormalities in the rectum and nearby structures, including the prostate. Also called endorectal ultrasound and ERUS.

Transurethral resection of the prostate (TRANZ-yooREE-thrul ree-SEK-shun...PROS-tayt): TURP. A surgical procedure to remove tissue from the prostate using an instrument inserted through the urethra.

Triptorelin (trip-toh-REL-in): A drug that is used to treat advanced prostate cancer and is being studied in the treatment of breast cancer. It belongs to the family of hormonal drugs called gonadotropin-releasing hormone analogs. Also called Trelstar.

Tumor (TOO-mer): An abnormal mass of tissue that results when cells divide more than they should or do not die when they should. Tumors may be benign (not cancerous) or malignant (cancerous). Also called neoplasm.

Ultrasound (UL-truh-SOWND): A procedure in which high-energy sound waves (ultrasound) are bounced off internal tissues or organs and make echoes. The echo patterns are shown on the screen of an ultrasound machine, forming a picture of body tissues called a sonogram. Also called ultrasonography.

Urethra (yoo-REE-thruh): The tube through which urine leaves the body. It empties urine from the bladder.

Urinary incontinence (YOOR-in-air-ee in-KAHN-tihnens): Inability to hold urine in the bladder.

Urologic oncologist (YOOR-uh-LAH-jik on-KAH-lojist): A doctor who specializes in treating cancers of the urinary system.

Urologist (yoo-RAH-loh-jist): A doctor who specializes in diseases of the urinary organs in females and the urinary and sex organs in males.

Vaccine : A substance or group of substances meant to cause the immune system to respond to a tumor or to microorganisms, such as bacteria or viruses. A vaccine can help the body recognize and destroy cancer cells or microorganisms.

Vasectomy (va-SEK-toh-mee): An operation to cut or tie off the two tubes that carry sperm out of the testicles.

Vitamin E: A substance used in cancer prevention. It belongs to the family of drugs called tocopherols.

Watchful waiting : Closely monitoring a patient's condition but withholding treatment until symptoms appear or change. Also called observation.

X-ray : A type of high-energy radiation. In low doses, x-rays are used to diagnose diseases by making pictures of the inside of the body. In high doses, x-rays are used to treat cancer.

National Cancer Institute Information Resources 50 National Cancer Institute Publications

You may want more information for yourself, your family, and your doctor. The following NCI services are available to help you.

Telephone

NCI's Cancer Information Service (CIS) provides accurate, up-to-date information about cancer to patients and their families, health professionals, and the general public. Information specialists translate the latest scientific information into plain language, and they will respond in English or Spanish, as well as through TRS providers for the hearing or speech impaired. Calls to the CIS are confidential and free.

Telephone: 1–800–4–CANCER (1–800–422–6237)
Internet

NCI's Web site provides information from numerous NCI sources. It offers current information about cancer prevention, screening, diagnosis, treatment, genetics, supportive care, and ongoing clinical trials. It has information about NCI's research programs, funding opportunities, and cancer statistics.

Web site: http://www.cancer.gov
Spanish Web site: http://www.cancer.gov/espanol

If you're unable to find what you need on the Web site, contact NCI staff. Use the online contact form at http://www.cancer.gov/contact or send an email to cancer-govstaff@mail.nih.gov.

Also, information specialists provide live, online assistance through LiveHelp at
http://www.cancer.gov/help.

National Cancer Institute Publications

NCI provides publications about cancer, including the booklets and fact sheets mentioned in this booklet. Many are available in both English and Spanish.

You may order these publications by telephone, on the Internet, or by mail. You may also read them online and print your own copy.

• By telephone: People in the United States and its territories may order these and other NCI publications by calling the NCI's Cancer

Information Service at 1–800–4–CANCER.

• On the Internet: Many NCI publications may be viewed, downloaded, and ordered from

http://www.cancer.gov/publications on the Internet. People in the United States and its territories may use this Web site to order printed copies. This Web site also explains how people outside the United States can mail or fax their requests for NCI booklets.

• By mail: NCI publications may be ordered by writing to the address below:

Publications Ordering Service

National Cancer Institute

P.O. Box 24128

Baltimore, MD 21227

PSA Test and Prostate Changes

• The Prostate-Specific Antigen (PSA) Test: Questions and Answers

• Understanding Prostate Changes: A Health Guide for Men

Prostate Cancer

• Treatment Choices for Men with Early-Stage Prostate Cancer

• Early Prostate Cancer: Questions and Answers

- What You Need To Know About™ Prostate Cancer (also in Spanish)
Clinical Trials

- Taking Part in Cancer Treatment Research Studies
Finding a Doctor, Support Groups, or Other Organizations

- How To Find a Doctor or Treatment Facility If You Have Cancer (also in Spanish)
- Cancer Support Groups: Questions and Answers
- National Organizations That Offer Services to People With Cancer and Their Families (also in Spanish)

Cancer Treatment and Supportive Care

- Radiation Therapy and You (also in Spanish)
- Understanding Radiation Therapy: What To Know About External Beam Radiation Therapy (also in Spanish)

- Understanding Radiation Therapy: What To Know About Brachytherapy (A Type of Internal Radiation Therapy) (also in Spanish)

- Chemotherapy and You (also in Spanish)

National Cancer Institute Information Resources 50 National Cancer Institute Publications

• Cryosurgery in Cancer Treatment: Questions and Answers

• Eating Hints for Cancer Patients (also in Spanish)

• Pain Control (also in Spanish)

Coping with Cancer

• Taking Time: Support for People with Cancer

• Managing Radiation Therapy Side Effects: What Men Can Do About Changes in Sexuality and Fertility Side Effects (also in Spanish)

• Managing Radiation Therapy Side Effects: What To Do About Changes When You Urinate (also in Spanish)

• Managing Radiation Therapy Side Effects: What To Do When You Feel Weak or Tired (Fatigue) (also in Spanish)

Life After Cancer Treatment

• Facing Forward: Life After Cancer Treatment (also in Spanish)

• Follow-up Care After Cancer Treatment: Questions and Answers

• Facing Forward: Ways You Can Make a Difference in Cancer

Advanced or Recurrent Cancer

- Coping With Advanced Cancer
- When Cancer Returns

Complementary Medicine

- Thinking about Complementary & Alternative Medicine: A guide for people with cancer
- Complementary and Alternative Medicine in Cancer Treatment: Questions and Answers (also in Spanish)

Caregivers

- When Someone You Love Is Being Treated for Cancer: Support for Caregivers
- When Someone You Love Has Advanced Cancer: Support for Caregivers
- Facing Forward: When Someone You Love Has Completed Cancer Treatment
- Caring for the Caregiver: Support for Cancer Caregivers

NIH Publication No. 08-1576 Revised September 2008 Printed September 2008